VALUABLE HERBAL PRESCRIPTIONS

VARIOUS AILMENTS AND THEIR TREATMENT BY NATURE'S REMEDIES

First Edition 1895
Bradford Medical Institute

New Edition 2017

Edited by Tarl Warwick
Illustrated by Rita Metzner

1

COPYRIGHT AND DISCLAIMER

FOREWORD

This following text was apparently released by the Bradford Medical Institute of Yorkshire. It is one part herbal, one part pharmaceutical literature of its age, and every part a quack work of sorts- for while herbal compounds may indeed have significant effects on human health, some of the suggested cures and treatments here are badly dated.

Perhaps this simplistic guide (richly illustrated as it is) is best seen in a historical light as the typical pre-modern prescriptive guide from its era. Such works were released generally in the late 19th century by pharmaceutical firms as prescription literature, or by individuals as *family physics*. The former often came with numerous ads for various tonics and pills, although this is mostly absent from the present work, to its credit.

Herbal medicine is of great interest within a spiritual context; we have today a rather large movement backwards to this essential era as truly modern medicine grapples with modern homeopathy and alternative medicine on one end, and its very real and potentially disastrous inability to deal with mutated viruses and bacteria on the other.

This edition of "Valuable Herbal Prescriptions" has been re-illustrated and edited for grammar and format. Care has been taken to retain original intent and meaning.

HERBAL PRESCRIPTIONS

Extract from Speech made at Guy's Hospital, London, March 26th, 1890.

"The origin of the medical profession was traceable to two sources- the first was the observation of nature which produced the herbalist... He was not aware whether botany now formed a recognized branch of medical education. He could not help wishing it did, because not only was it in itself a most beautiful and interesting study, exercising the mind without fatiguing it, and stimulating the imagination without leading it astray, but it led to a careful observation of nature, and to a habit of noticing the qualities of plants which were so remarkable and so powerful in their healing capacity. Perhaps his hearers would think it almost ludicrous if he told a little anecdote of his own, which, simple and slight though it was, still it illustrated what he meant. As was pretty well known, he had been given to the pursuit of wood-cutting. By pure accident he drew his finger one day along a tolerably sharp bit of the edge of his ax, and cut his finger. On searching about him he found he had no pocket handkerchief available. He wanted to staunch his little wound. He got a leaf and put it on. He was bound to say that it was not the result of botanical knowledge; it was strictly an empirical proceeding. But the curious result was that the healing of this little breach of continuity occupied exactly half the time unassisted nature would have required. It was perhaps hardly worth mentioning, but he could not help thinking that there were great treasures in nature more than had heretofore been explored in that as in every other branch."

-Daily News, March 27th, 1890.

HERBAL PRESCRIPTIONS

I can readily confirm the above statement; there is scarcely a plant that grows, but which, on being analyzed, will be found to contain certain medicinal properties, which if properly applied, would have a beneficial influence upon the ailment for which it is adapted. For instance, certain plants act as purgatives, some as emetics, some induce perspiration, others expectoration, some act upon the kidneys, some upon the liver, whilst others act upon the salivary glands, the blood, skin, nerve tissues, etc; and when a compound is compounded of harmless vegetable ingredients, may be taken for any length of time, and nothing but good will attend their use; and when they have done their work will leave the system all the better for it; such cannot always be said of minerals, of mercury never. There are many preparations I could select for the various ailments named in this book, but I confine myself to those given, in consequence of their general effectiveness during long and varied experience. In September, 1882, I received the following (unsolicited) letter from the Right Hon. W. E Gladstone :

> 10, Downing Street,
> Whitehall,
> London.
> Sept. 28th, 1882.
>
> Sir,
>
> I am directed by Mr. Gladstone to thank you for recommending the cure for Catarrh. I am, Sir, Your obedient servant.
>
> -G. Leveson-Gower.

Using letters from grateful patients is not a weakness of mine, but I publish this because of the Right Hon. gentleman's speech; and if time, space, and the weakness, would permit, I could publish a list of testimonials every week all the year round. But the price of a trial of the Prescriptions given in this book is so paltry that no ailing person can form a reasonable excuse for not testing their virtue; besides, I do not pretend that the remedies are infallible, there is no such thing as an infallible remedy, to make the assertion means quackery; but I do assert that they are well worth a trial, and if you or yours fare as well as the majority you will have little to complain of, and much to be grateful for.

I am continually receiving letters asking questions on the subject of physical culture as a curative agent, the following is my opinion:

Physical Culture will make the strong stronger.

Physical Culture would be beneficial to people of sedentary occupation.

Physical Culture cannot cure disease.

Physical Culture cannot take the place of medicine.

Physical Culture injudiciously indulged in can do much injury.

Weight-lifting is not an advisable pastime, it may be all right for a man of herculean strength who knows himself master of the weights he is going to handle, but for the average man this occupation can only be attended with much danger of producing rupture. No man even at his work should attempt to lift anything he thinks is beyond his strength, he will act wisely in asking a mate to give him a hand. People whose employment is laborious (or fairly active) need no physical exercise.

HERBAL PRESCRIPTIONS

RHEUMATISM

The joints and muscles are the parts affected, the movement of the same causing pain, in severe cases the joints swell and become very much inflamed. When in the joints it is described simply as Rheumatism or Rheumatics, when in the muscles it is described as Muscular Rheumatism.

Causes: Taking alcoholic drinks to excess, getting the clothes wet through, sleeping in damp beds, lying on damp grass, getting one cold on top of another, etc.

Treatment: Have a vapor or Turkish bath every week if possible, and guard against chill. Prepare the following:

Agrimony ½ oz
Bogbean ½ oz
Raspberry Leaves ½ oz
Arcticum Lappa ½ oz
Achilloe Millefolium, the herb ½ oz

Boil in a quart of water slowly for 5 minutes, strain, and when cold take a wineglass full three times a day; and at bedtime take a pill of the following:

Lobelia Herb 2 drachms.
Gum Arabic 2 drachms.
Capsicum 1 drachm.

Mix with Gum Mucilage, and make into 4 grain pills. Dose: One pill at bedtime.

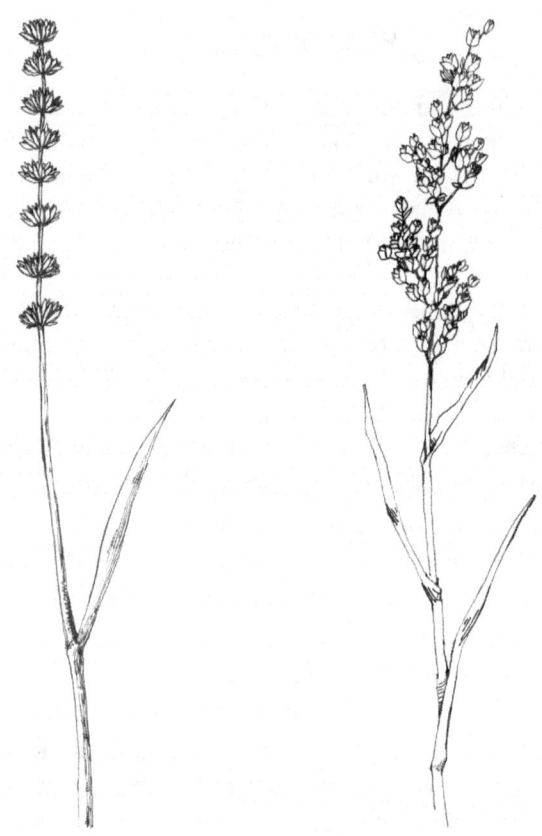

Dog's Grass & Australian Field Grass

SCIATICA

Causes: Taking cold, general debility, impaired vitality, etc.

Symptoms: Acute pain in the hip, and sometimes extending from the hip to the knee, in advanced cases extending to the foot. It is sometimes tedious of cure.

Treatment:

Populus Tremuloids, the bark 1 oz
Juniper Berries 1 oz
Myrica Cerifera ½ oz
Ginger ½ oz

Boil in a quart of water (slowly) for 5 minutes, strain, and when cold take a wineglass full 3 or 4 times a day. The medicine must be kept in a cold place.

Lotion:

Spirits of Hartshorn 1 oz
Sweet Oil 1 oz
Tincture of Myrrh 1 oz

Shake well the Bottle and gently but perseveringly rub into the affected parts twice a day.

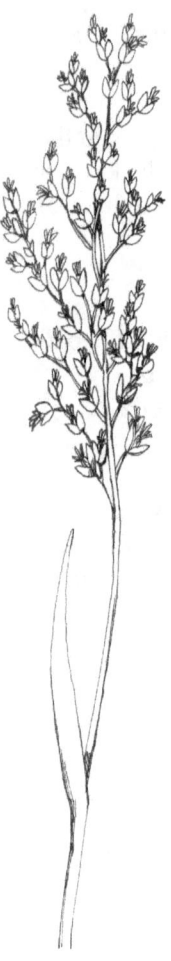

Holy Grass

PERMISO

HERBAL PRESCRIPTIONS

KIDNEY AND BLADDER TROUBLE

Symptoms: Heaviness, drowsiness, pains at the bottom of the back, sometimes a shooting pain, at other times a dull pain, dizziness in the head, variable action of the heart, scanty urine with frequent desire to pass same, etc. When dropsical swellings take place the disease is advanced, and is then styled Bright's Disease. Eat sparingly; let your diet be plain but substantial; avoid that mentioned later in this work.

Treatment:

Dog's Grass ½ oz
Pellitory of the Wall ½ oz
Clivers ½ oz
Juniperus Communis, the berry ½ oz
Alchemilla Arvensis ½ oz

Boil slowly in a quart of water 5 minutes, strain, and when cold take a wineglass full 3 or 4 times a day, indulge as much in open air as possible. The medicine must be kept in a cold place.

One pill at bedtime. The same pill as for Nervous Debility, shall be given.

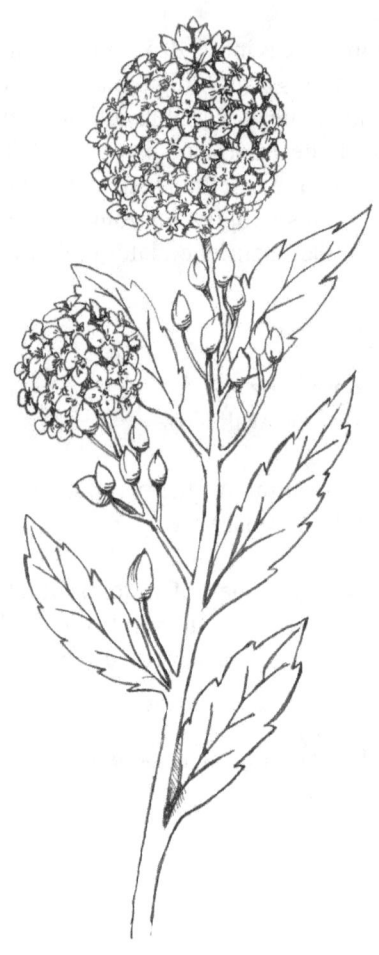

Maritima

HERBAL PRESCRIPTIONS

SORE EYES

Keep the eyelids clean, and night and morning foment the same a minute or so with equal parts milk and water, warm; and afterwards rub in gently a little of the following ointment:

Ointment:

White Wax 1 oz
Olive Oil 2 drachms
Mutton Suet 2 drachms
Oil of Roses 1 drachm

Melt the mutton suet and wax, add the oil and roses, and stir until cold.

If vitiated blood be the cause take also the following medicine:

Rubus Strigosus, the leaves 1 oz
Galium Aperine ½ oz
Ground Ivy ½ oz
Child's Powder ½ oz

Boil in a quart of water slowly for 3 minutes, strain, and when cold take a wineglass full 3 times a day. The medicine must be kept in a cold place. It may be sweetened with sugar if desired; dose for children must be reduced accordingly. Open air exercise should be indulged in as much as possible. Inherited sore eyes can seldom be cured, but even in these cases this treatment should prove very beneficial.

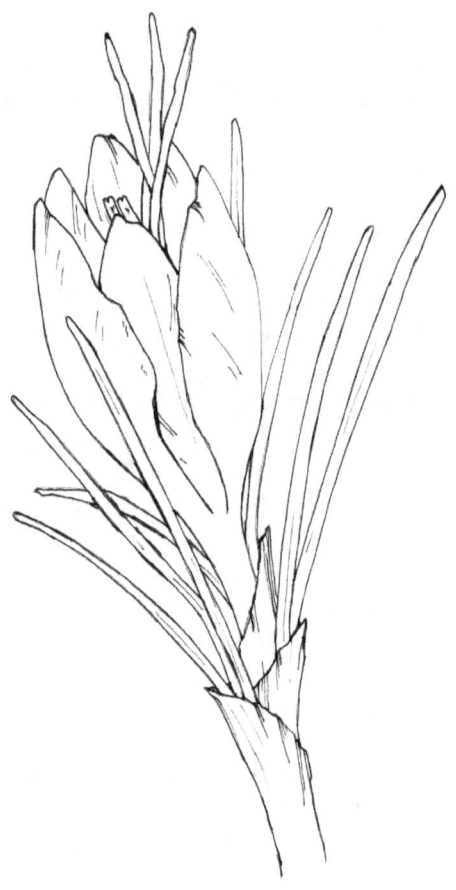

Saffron

HERBAL PRESCRIPTIONS

ULCERATED THROAT

Causes: Working or living in an impure atmosphere, unwholesome food, neglected cleanliness, etc.

Treatment:

Agrimony ½ oz
Raspberry leaves ½ oz
Galium Aperine ½ oz
Gentian root ½ oz
Cassia ½ oz

Boil in a quart of water slowly for 3 minutes, strain, and when cold take a wine glass full three times a day. The medicine must be kept in a cold place.

Gargle: 1 part tincture of myrrh to 7 parts water, and add 15 drops tincture of cayenne; with this gargle the throat 3 or 4 times a day, and keep the bowels nice and regular if not already so.

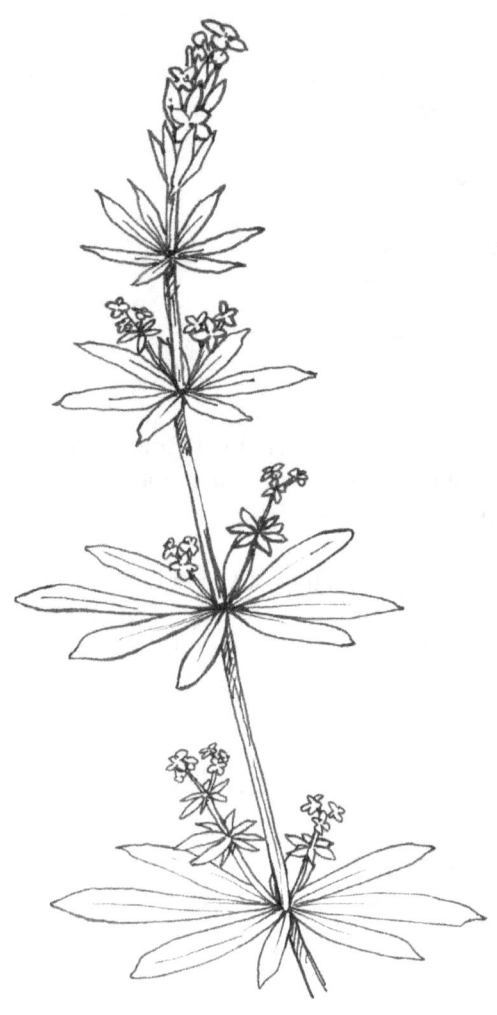

Galium Aperine

ULCERATED STOMACH

Causes: Long continued stomach derangement, unwholesome food, debility, excess in alcohol drinking, etc.

Symptoms: Dull heavy sensation at the pit of the stomach, occasional swelling of the same with occasional cramp feeling, sickly feeling with sometimes a tendency to vomit, restlessness and variable pulse, depressed in spirit, temporary absence of strength, if the disease be advanced the tongue also becomes somewhat ulcerated.

Treatment:

Clivers ½ oz
Arctium Lappa, the root ½ oz
Raspberry Leaves ½ oz

Boil in a quart of water (slowly) for 5 minutes, strain, fill up to a quart and when cold take a wineglass full 3 or 4 times a day. The medicine must be kept in a cold place. And at bedtime 2 pills composed as follows:

Solid Extract Cascara 2 drachms
Capsicum 1 drachm
Extract of Chamomilla 2 drachms

Mix with Gum Mucilage. Make into 4 grain pills.

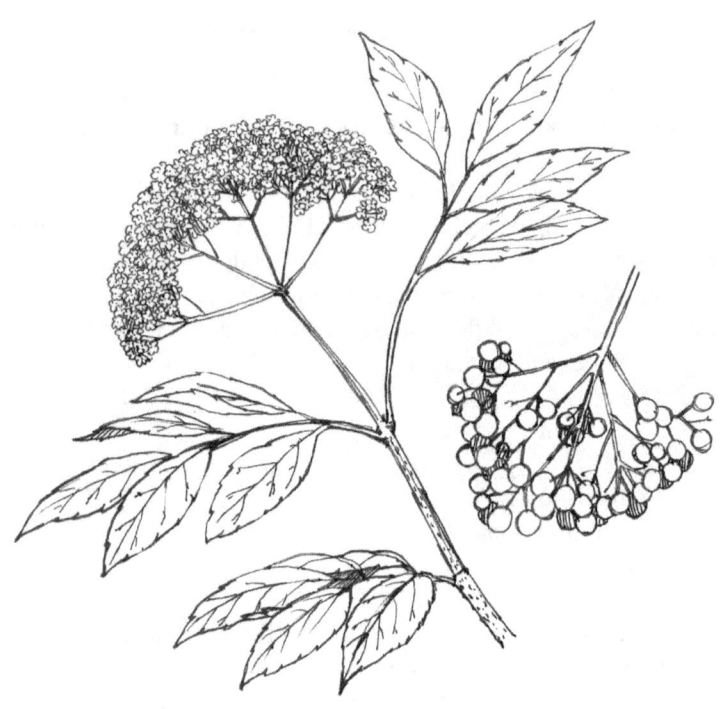

Elder

HEADACHE

Causes: The causes are too numerous to mention: constipation, obstructed blood circulation in the head, overeating, brain worry, disordered stomach, etc; in females obstruction of the menses is a common cause.

Treatment

Scullcap ½ oz
Rosemary ½ oz
Taraxacum, the herb ½ oz
Menthe Viride ½ oz
Verbena Herb 1 oz

Boil slowly in a quart of water 3 minutes, strain, and when cold take a wineglass full three times a day. The medicine must be kept in a cold place.

Keep the bowels nicely regular with the following pills:

Solid Extract Cascara 2 drachms
Lobelia Herb 2 drachms
Turkey Rhubarb 2 drachms
Extract of Dock 2 drachms

Form into pill mass, make into 4 grain pills.

Dose: One or two pills at bedtime three nights a week. Indulge in open air as much as possible, and also follow instructions in bedroom ventilating (if possible.)

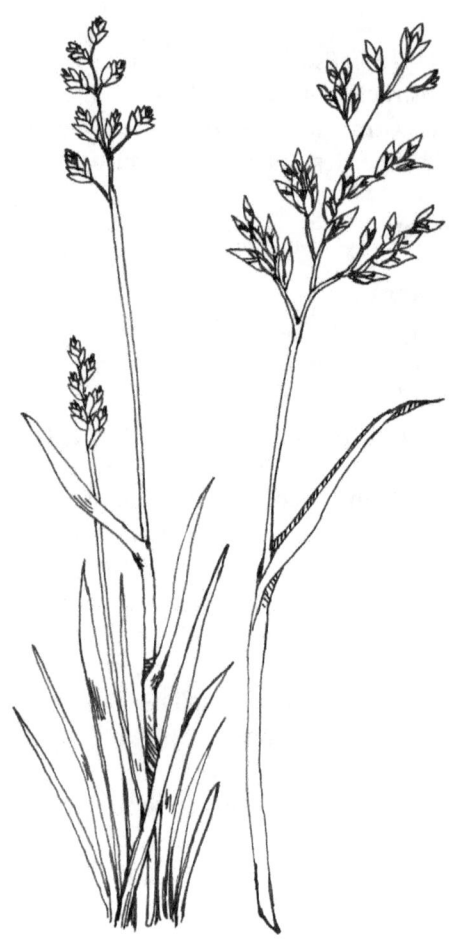

Foreign Grasses

HERBAL PRESCRIPTIONS

NERVOUS DEBILITY (Constitutional)

Nervous debility is so well known that it scarcely needs describing, and shows itself in a dozen different ways. Fears (groundless), tremors, dread of coming evil, lack of courage, startled at the least unexpected sound, buzzing noises in the head, ringing in the head, restlessness, shy of company, lacking confidence in one's everyday work; in advanced cases trembling (or shakiness) of the hands, etc; at the commencement of the ailment one or two of the symptoms only may be present, followed by the rest as the debility advances.

Treatment:

skullcap ½ oz
Mistletoe ½ oz
Menyanthes ½ oz
Gentian ½ oz

Boil in a quart of water slowly for 5 minutes, strain, and when cold take a wine glass full 3 times a day. The medicine must be kept in a cold place.

Pills as follows:

Lobelia herb 2 drachms
Gum arabic 2 drachms
Capsicum 1 drachm

Mix with gum mucilage and make into 4 grain pills. Dose; 1 pill at bedtime.

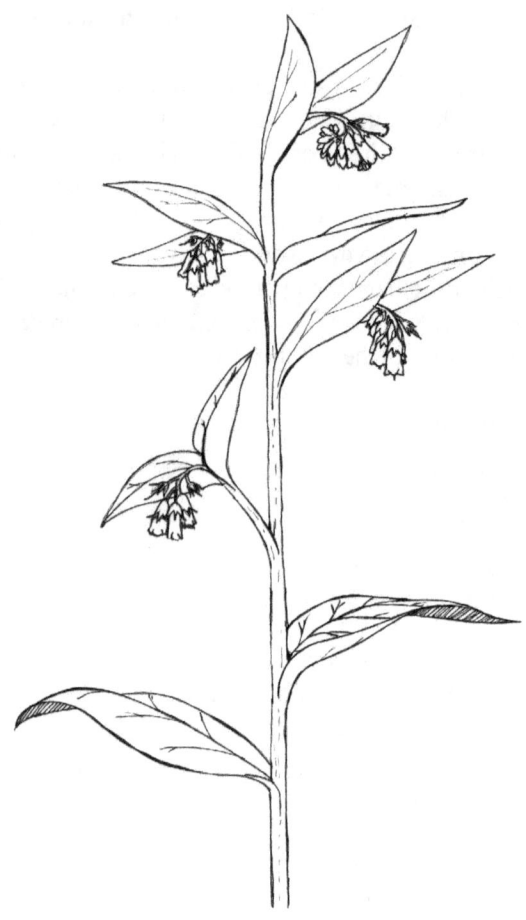

Comfrey

HERBAL PRESCRIPTIONS

BLOOD DISEASES (Constitutional)

Causes: Living in thickly populated districts, closely confined rooms, working in vitiated atmosphere, free use of malt alcohol, eating tainted food; it is sometimes left in the train of scarlet fever, measles, etc., and is often inherited.

Symptoms: The symptoms are too well known and too numerous to need describing.

Treatment:

Sassafras Bark ½ oz
Achilloe ½ oz
Sarsaparilla ½ oz
Arctium Lappa ½ oz
Galium Aperine ½ oz
Guiacum Raspings ½ oz
Astragalus (the root) 6 drachms

Boil the lot in a quart of water slowly for 15 minutes, then strain, boil the same a second time in a pint of water 5 minutes, strain, add to the other, and when cold add the juice of a large lemon, and take a large wineglass full (or a half-tumblerful) three times a day. Keep this medicine in a cold place. Sponge the body with equal parts vinegar and cold water, rub briskly until thoroughly dry with a coarse bath towel, this may be done every other day if possible, it is not absolutely necessary but highly beneficial. A vegetable diet is good, also lean beef, lean mutton, or fish; avoid fat, coffee, cheese, pork, stew, sausage, all highly seasoned dishes, jams, and pickles. When procurable an occasional Turkish bath is highly beneficial. Spend plenty of lime in the cooling room and guard against chill on leaving the baths.

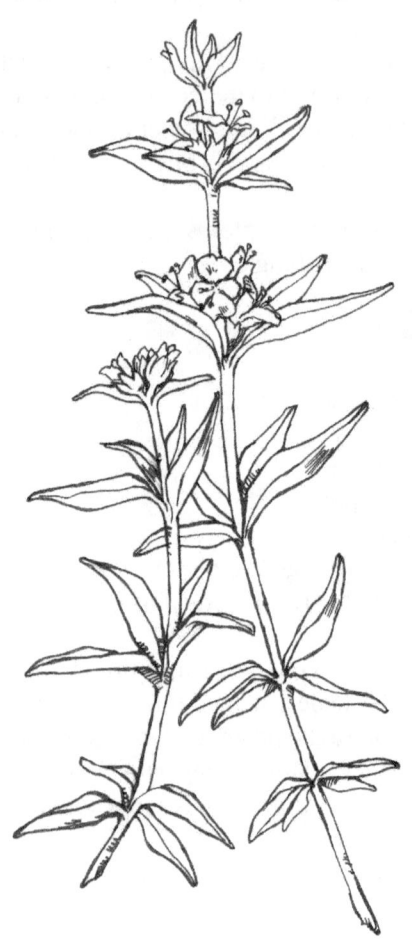

Hyssop

HERBAL PRESCRIPTIONS

PILES

Piles come under two classes, bleeding and blind. There are numerous causes; wine drinking, excessive purging with pills containing aloes, pills containing mercury, highly seasoned food, thoughtlessly sitting on cold or damp stone, etc. In others the disease is inherited, in inherited cases there is no certainty of a permanent cure, when cured it is liable to return at any time.

Treatment:

Pile Powder 1 oz
Honey 4 oz

Mix into a soft paste and take a teaspoonful 4 or 5 times a day.

Boil 1 oz. Marshmallow Root in a quart of Milk slowly for two minutes (carefully watch it or it will instantly boil over and you will lose the lot), drink freely of this as often as you please; if too cloggy composed of all milk, use equal parts milk and water; this must be kept in a cold place. Night and morning wash the seat (anus) and sponge a few minutes with cold water, dry with a cloth, and gently but perseveringly rub in a little Pile Ointment composed of Gall.

Keep the bowels easy with turkey rhubarb advised for constipation.

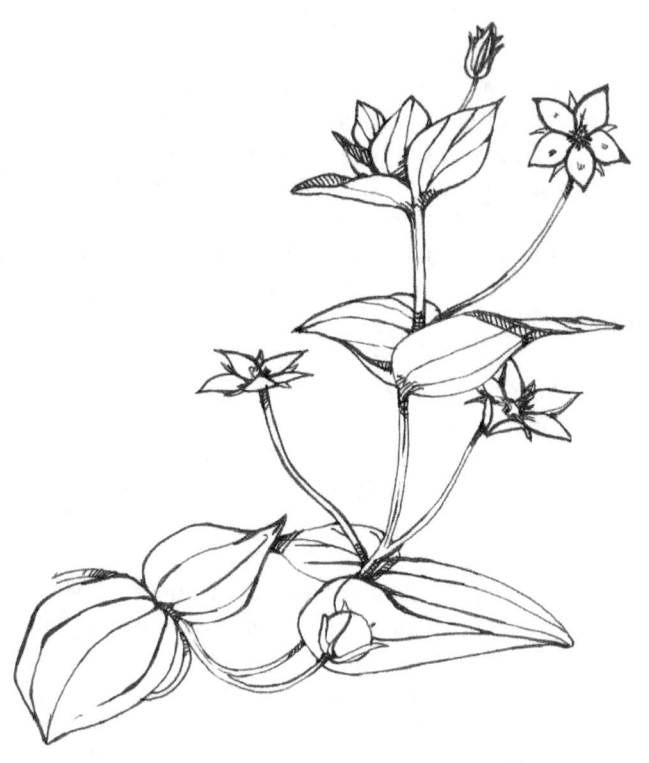

Pimpernel

HERBAL PRESCRIPTIONS

LIVER AFFECTIONS

This disease shows itself in many different forms, with some people the symptoms are very prominent, whilst in others very obscure; there are numerous causes. Symptoms: Sallow complexion, languidness, variable appetite, depression of spirits, sometimes constipated, at others a kind of prickly purge; when the white of the eye is a yellow tint the ailment is advanced.

Treatment: Eat sparingly, do not overload your stomach, let your diet be plain and simple, avoid all kinds of highly seasoned dishes, stews, cheese, pork, jam, pastry, pickles, and all kinds of sweets. Indulge in open air as much as possible, and if in the habit of taking intoxicants let them rest for 6 or 8 weeks.

Taraxacum Root ½ oz
Myrica Cerifera ½ oz
Agrimony ½ oz
Hydrastis Canadensis ½ oz
Stomach Bitters (powder) a half teaspoonful.

Boil in a quart of water slowly for 5 minutes, strain, and when cold take a wineglass full 3 times a day. This medicine must be kept in a cold place. The following Pills are very valuable in helping the cure:

Gentiana Lutea 2 drachms
Lobelia Herb 2 drachms
Taraxacum 2 drachms
Golden Seal 4 drachms

Mix into pill mass with Gum Mucilage, make into 3 grain pills. Dose: One pill twice a day immediately after meals.

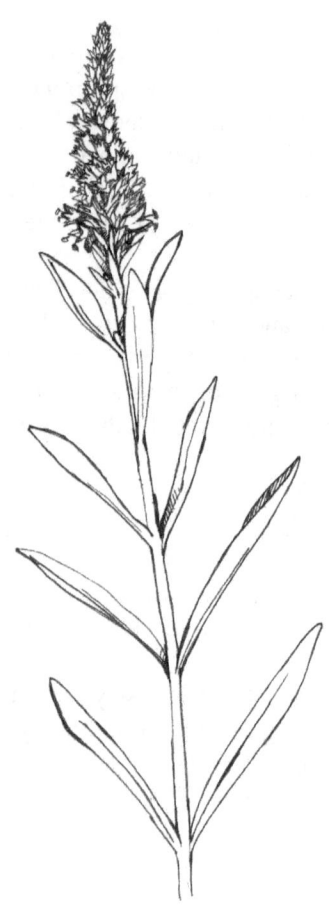

Speedwell

LUMBAGO

Symptoms: In some instances kidney trouble could easily be mistaken for lumbago, as also rheumatism, but the most pointed symptoms of lumbago are, when rising from a sitting position, there is much difficulty in straightening one's self, with sometimes a dull pain in trying to do so, pains at the bottom of the back in the region of the kidneys.

Cause: It mostly arises from chill, or repeated chills (colds) in the back.

Treatment:

Juniper berries ½ oz
Tanacetum Vulgare ½ oz
Uva ursi ½ oz
Bog bean ½ oz
Caulophyllum 1 drachm

Boil very slowly for 5 minutes in a quart of water, strain, and when cold take a wineglass full 3 times a day. This medicine must be kept in a cold place.

The following pill may be taken at bedtime:

Lobelia herb 2 drachms
Gum arabic 2 drachms
Capsicum 1 drachm

Mix with gum mucilage and form into 4 grain pills.

GRAVEL AND STONE

Causes: Excess in alcohol, especially fermented wines, rich diet, inactivity, drinking well water, etc.

Symptoms: Sickness, sometimes a desire to vomit, disturbed urine, sometimes tinged with blood, red deposit sticking to bottom of chamber utensil after urine, sometimes gritty, occasional pain extending to the bladder, sometimes swelling of the leg or thigh, difficulty in passing urine, etc.

Stone: Urinary obstruction, sometimes passing very small pebbles, dribbling urine, occasional pains at the bladder neck, at times thick, milky looking urine with very strong smell.

Treatment:

Pellitory of the Wall ½ oz
Gravel Root ½ oz
Parsley Peirt ½ oz
Achilloe ½ oz
Wintergreen ½ oz
Althoea ½ oz

Boil in a quart of water slowly for 5 minutes, strain, and add to the hot liquid 2 oz. of honey, mix well. Dose when cold: A wineglass full 3 times a day. This medicine must be kept in a cold place.

HERBAL PRESCRIPTIONS

If the bowels are not nicely regular a 3 grain pill at bedtime composed as follows may be taken:

> Extract of Taraxacum 1 drachm
> Turkey Rhubarb 2 drachms
> Oil of Menthe Viride 10 drops

Form into pill mass and divide into 3 grain pills.

Dose: One pill at bedtime 2 or 3 nights a week.

BLACKHEADS

Blackheads, commonly called grubs, should be gently squeezed out as they appear; always wash in water with the chill taken off (never really cold water) and use a coarse flannel to wash with sulfate of zinc ointment is as good as anything that can be used.

PIMPLES

There are many varieties of pimples, but all that need concern the patient are the two kinds which may be described as the soft and the hard, the soft ripen and fill with a cream tinted matter which can be pricked with a needle and the matter gently squeezed out, it then dries up and disappears; the other kind do not contain matter and might justly be described as skin eruptions; both kinds are constitutional, that is to say not a disease; the same may be said of blackheads and acne. There are few cases which can be permanently cured, they are liable to return at any time. Zinc lotion or zinc ointment will do all for them that can be done.

ACNE

Acne spots might justly be described as choked up perspiration, and need precisely the same treatment as for Blackheads.

A small bottle of zinc lotion can be procured at any chemist's for a few coppers. Zinc ointment in penny, two penny or three penny tins. Those really desirous of trying an internal treatment cannot adopt anything better than the medicine for Blood disease, see prior, but as previously stated there is no certainty as to the cure being permanent.

GASTRIC TROUBLE

Symptoms: Food turning to acid bile, or acid gas, heaviness and sluggishness until it passes away; sometimes gas fumes rise into the throat or mouth.

Cause: Indigestion.

Treatment:

Hydrastin 32 grains
Xanthoxylin 32 grains
Avenin 32 grains
Sodi Bicarb 160 grains
Water to 4 ounces

Dose: A teaspoonful in a wineglass of water three times a day, soon after each meal. Also follow bedroom ventilation (if possible) and diet.

HERBAL PRESCRIPTIONS

ACIDITYOF THE STOMACH - BILIOUSNESS

Much akin to the above named, same treatment. Open air as much as possible, and walking exercise considerably helps the cure of the above; also see diet particulars.

WATERBRASH

Symptoms: Clear liquid (waterlike) and of an acid taste rising into the mouth after eating a little cheese, an unripe apple, or anything of a nondigestive nature; it is mostly found in young people.

The following simple things will usually counteract the acid; crush a piece of school chalk under the blade of a knife, crush it into a fine powder, put as much as would cover a shilling on the tongue and wash it down with a little milk and water. Another simple counteraction is a pinch of salt in a quarter of a glass of milk, fill up the glass with hot water and slowly drink it.

FITS

Loss of the senses, followed by inward convulsions, but the symptoms are so well known both by the afflicted and the non-afflicted that it is useless to dwell on them.

Cause: The causes are numerous, the most frequent being injury to the back of the head by falling or otherwise; run down constitution, nerve troubles, or anything which diminishes vitality.

Treatment:

Tanacetum (the herb) ½ oz
Pellitory of the Wall ½ oz
Leonurus Cardiaca ½ oz
Mistletoe ½ oz
Rue ½ oz

Boil in a quart of water slowly for five minutes, strain, and when cold take a wineglass full three times a day This medicine must be kept in a cold place. And the following pills at bedtime:

Lobelia Extract 2 drachms
Asafoetida Extract 2 drachms

Form into 4 grain pills and take two every night.

Sponging the body three times a week with equal parts vinegar and cold water, afterwards rubbing briskly until thoroughly dry with a coarse bath towel would be very helpful.

Also follow instructions as to ventilated bedroom.

INDIGESTION

I have always maintained that indigestion is incurable, and have not yet had cause to alter my opinion. When people tell me that I or anyone else have cured them of indigestion, I know that they never really had it, and by close questioning usually find that they had cured themselves of excessive eating; that by reducing the quantity of food they were in the habit of consuming they had assisted the stomach in performing its proper functions.

HERBAL PRESCRIPTIONS

These cases cannot be described as indigestion in the true sense of the term, they might justly be described as overtaxed stomachs; there is a vast difference between an overtaxed stomach and indigestion, the former will perform its functions if not overtaxed, without medicine, but the latter would also need medicinal aid; or to describe it more accurately we might call the former an abused stomach, not a non-digestive stomach. The nondigestive stomach is the real source of trouble, a stomach not up to much when at its best, whether studying diet or not, and herein lies the true definition of the word Indigestion. Another remarkable thing connected with indigestion is there is no rule as to diet. The writer of this book having all his life had to study his diet must be allowed to know a little on this subject, few people having tried more remedies, and although he never met with that infallible cure one reads of in the newspapers, he is still living, with little to complain of, and long life is what we seek to attain.

There never was nor ever will be an infallible cure for indigestion. The food which would digest with one person would fail to digest with another, and the best means to adopt is to take particular notice of the kind of food which best agrees with you and keep to it, allowing your stomach to be the judge. The same may almost be said of medicines, but I recommend the two prescriptions here appended, because of their general effectiveness during a long and varied experience.

Causes: Impaired vitality, overloading the stomach, worry, excess of brain work, closely confined rooms, sedentary occupation, spitting whilst tobacco smoking, excessive drinking of ardent spirits, in fact excess in any kind of alcohol; whilst a large number inherit this defect.

Symptoms: The symptoms are numerous, the following being only a few. A sense of heaviness in the stomach, sometimes attended with a dull pain, a feeling of sluggishness soon after meals, occasional sensations of dizziness in the head, heart palpitation; certain kinds of food will turn to acid, belching of wind, flatulence. If allowed to continue unassisted the person becomes a confirmed dyspeptic, hypochondriac, etc. in progressive cases only one or two symptoms may be observed, whilst in advanced cases many, and in old standing cases the lot. Proceed as follows :

Eat slowly of the food which you know from experience best agrees with you; if you have not taken notice of this, take notice. Always cease eating when you could eat a little more; you do not benefit from the large quantity eaten, the true benefit is derived from the reasonable quantity digested. You may with advantage avoid the following; cheese, pork, stews, hash, sausage, all kinds of highly seasoned dishes, pickles, and jams.

Treatment:

Agrimony ½ oz
Raspberry Leaves ½ oz
Galium Aperine ½ oz
Centarium ½ oz
Stomach Bitters (powder) ½ teaspoonfull.

Boil slowly in a quart of water 3 minutes, strain, and when cold take a wineglass full 3 times a day. This medicine must be kept in a cold place. Also take the following digestive pills:

Lobelia Herb 2 drachms
Capsicum ½ oz
Turkey Rhubarb ½ oz
Caryuphyllus ½ oz

HERBAL PRESCRIPTIONS

Form into pill mass with Extract of Gentian, make into 4 grain pills, and take one pill 3 times a day with each meal, immediately after meals. These pills (apart from the herb medicine) answer for many people, consequently a shilling box could be sent without the herbs. Also follow the open air particulars on, and the bedroom ventilation instructions.

CONSUMPTION, BRONCHITIS AND ASTHMA CURE

Prescription:

Marshmallow Root 2 drachms
Licorice Root 2 drachms
English Linseed ½ oz
Iceland Moss ½ oz
Hydrastis Canadensis 2 drachms
Life Root 2 drachms
Pleurisy Root 2 drachms

Directions: Place the whole of the ingredients into two pints of cold water and simmer or boil slowly for 5 minutes, occasionally stirring; whilst hot strain through a piece of muslin or fine sieve, then add and dissolve 2 oz. of sugar, or 10 pieces of lump sugar of ordinary size. If for a cough absolute, add double quantity of sugar and 2 tablespoonfuls of best vinegar. The sugar must not be added until the liquid is strained from the herbs. When cold fill up to a quart. The mixture must not be taken until cold; and must be kept in a cold place; and if bottled the bottle must be thoroughly cleaned after each making (for simple cough it may be taken warm).

Dose: A wineglass full three or four times a day, between meals if possible. This medicine must be kept in a cold place.

LOSSES BY WAR EXCEEDED

Extract. Daily Mail, January 25, 1900.

We grieve over the numerous brave men slain in the South African War, but their numbers, said a medical gentleman at a meeting of the Church Sanitary Association, held in the Westminster Palace Hotel, last night, are insignificant when compared with the number of those who, since the war began, have died in Great Britain of Consumption. No fewer than 20,000 persons have succumbed to the ravages of the deadly disease during the last four months. Considering the above remarkable statistics, perhaps my readers who have cause to dread the development of this dire disease would like a simple, inexpensive, and effective remedy in all cases where the lungs are not already diseased, even then its active principles will prolong life, and longevity is only what the best of us seek to attain; it will be found a winter's friend in chest and bronchial affections, including wheezing asthma, and all wasting disease.

We will send to any address in the kingdom a packet, post paid, of the above prescription on receipt of Postal Order for one shilling, or 12 penny stamps; three packets post paid for 2/9.

FALLING HAIR

As an outward application to arrest falling of the hair and to promote its growth, have the following made up at any first-class herbalists:

Cantharides 1 oz
Bay Rum ½ oz
Musk 2 drachms
Rosemary 2 drachms

HERBAL PRESCRIPTIONS

Water 4 oz

Shake well the bottle and rub a little into the roots of the hair once a day. This prescription is both harmless and effective.

CHILD'S CORDIAL

For disturbed sleep and gripes in children.

Lobelia Syrup 3 oz
Tincture of Valerian 2 drachms
Essence of Aniseed 1 drachm

Dose: A teaspoonful every two or three hours.

SOOTHING SYRUP

For green stools, looseness of the bowels and gripes in infants.

Rhubarb 2 oz.
Aniseed 1 oz
Marshmallow Root 1 oz

Boil in a quart of water for 5 minutes, strain clear, place the liquid again into the pan and add i lb. of lump sugar, boil slowly a minute or two, stirring the while, lift off the scum floating on the surface, allow it to stand until cold, then bottle.

Dose: A teaspoonful five or six times a day.

WHOOPING COUGH

Best Treacle ½ lb
Tincture of Lobelia 1 oz

HERBAL PRESCRIPTIONS

Aniseed Water 1 oz

Make the treacle hot, and whilst hot add the lobelia and aniseed water, and stir until cold.

Dose: A teaspoonful occasionally.

TROUBLESOME PERIODS

Treatment:

Matricaria (the herb) ½ oz
Rue ½ oz
Leonurus Cardiaca ½ oz
Wintergreen ½ oz

Boil in a quart of water (slowly) 5 minutes, strain, and when cold take a wineglass full 3 or 4 times a day. The medicine must be kept in a cold place. Take two pills at bedtime composed as follows :

Hiera Picra 2 drachms
Mentha Pulegium (Extract) 2 drachms

Make into 4 grain pills.

Ladies subject to troublesome periods can greatly alleviate their suffering by proceeding with the above treatment about three days before the time, and continuing the medicine until the close, one packet will serve the time.

CONSTIPATION

For constipation take as much of the best powdered Turkey Rhubarb as would cover a sixpence, dissolved in a little milk and water at bedtime every night; and the following morning on awakening drink a half-pint of hot water. To move the bowels by natural means is the object; pill purging, or any kind of purging, is injurious, and sure to make you more constipated afterwards. Turkey Rhubarb also cleanses the stomach, and with most people answers splendidly. A good way of ensuring the quality of the rhubarb would be to buy it in the root (in the piece) and powder it yourself, the simple nutmeg grater will answer the purpose. The dose may be increased or decreased as occasion demands (some people being much easier moved than others) but avoid purging.

GOUT (Rich Man's)

The rich man's gout in nine cases out of ten arises from excess of too rich food, wines, etc; the remedy would be to live on a plain diet for a few weeks, avoiding all kinds of wines, beer, and stout; an occasional drop of whiskey may be indulged in if desired, much open air, and walking exercise as soon as able.

An eminent Welsh doctor, regarding the rich man's gout, said; Live on sixpence a day and earn it, and you need not fear its return.

GOUT (Poor Man's)

The poor man's gout arises from too little, or too poor food, causing an impoverished state of the system; the remedy (were such possible) would be to exchange tables with the rich man, this (perhaps) not being possible the substitute is: Live well on good substantial food, the very best you can afford, with, if you can afford it, an occasional glass of good port wine, or Guinness's (harp label) stout.

DYSPEPSIA

The same treatment as for indigestion, dyspepsia being indigestion in an advanced stage.

NERVOUS BREAKDOWN

The same treatment as for nervous debility, the trouble in this instance being either more advanced, or taking place more suddenly, it is then described as nerve collapse.

LACK OF THOUGHT CONCENTRATION

The same as for nervous debility, the only difference being that this inability often takes place without any of the other symptoms named in nervous debility being present.

ANEMIA (Bloodlessness)

Anemia will be better known to the reader as poor blood, or bloodlessness, which through some unaccountable reason is more frequently found in females than in males, and may arise from various causes which have a tendency to debilitate the system; among which may be named closely confined workrooms, or closely-confined rooms of any kind, poor diet, the breathing of impure air, insufficient attention to keeping the pores of the skin open, and various other causes too numerous to mention.

This is why we see so many pale, weary, and debilitated parents, and in numerous cases, weak, puny offspring. One would hardly expect to find a strong healthy child born of weak, debilitated parents. Such is scarcely in accordance with the laws of nature. Healthy plants are not produced from inferior seed and poor soil, and it is impossible for strength to be born of weakness. When the blood in its richness is not up to its proper gravity, taking into consideration that the liver, kidneys, heart, lungs and brain must be fed with it, it sounds to sense that such organs must fail to perform their proper function; and when these organs do fail or are feeble in their action, the local symptoms following are too numerous to mention, and the patient invariably begins to treat the local symptoms. The cause of course (in the majority of cases) is entirely overlooked-consequently, if the cause be not attacked the field of advertised specifics have full play, and the afflicted look in the paper for the (so-called) specific for their particular class of symptom or symptoms, as the case may be, and no doubt the majority of these proprietary medicines are very good, and will stimulate the organs for which they are adapted, but fail to produce any permanent beneficial effect in cases where the remedy is not adapted to the cause; whereas had the organs he was treating been at fault, the medicine in question would justly be termed a specific, because its influence on these particular organs would perform a cure.

Therefore where the symptoms mentioned arise from poorness of blood, whilst the patient is battling with first one specific and then another the debility is gradually gaining ground, and eventually the nervous system begins to relax, and constitutional nervous debility eventually makes its appearance.

When the patient reaches this stage he or she of course begins to be low-spirited, moodiness and despondency are prominent, everything- even their daily routine of business- seems a trouble, and yet rest makes little difference. Eventually all the local symptoms attending a deranged system are prevalent, and one begins to think there is no one on earth so badly dealt with, whereas there are thousands just thinking similarly of themselves; and if this state of affairs is allowed to continue it is not so very long before the stomach becomes weakened, and incapacity for digesting the food takes place; and if allowed to continue, dyspepsia (swelling after meals), but swelling after meals only takes place when the debility of the digestive organs is of long standing. General debility implies much, and would cover a whole category of symptoms. It is styled general debility because the person may appear to be suffering with all the ailments that flesh is heir to, and yet an examination does not show a deficiency of any particular organ, hence it is termed general. There can be no general debility in a healthy person, and there are few unhealthy persons where the blood is rich, pure, and up to the proper standard. The blood is the life, and upon it depends the proper working of the principal functions of the body. The Germ Syrup enriches and forms new blood, and slowly but surely builds up the system; to prove this you only need to weigh the patient before and after treatment on the same scales.

GERM SYRUP

The GERM SYRUP is a feeder of the blood, nerve, bone, muscle, flesh and tissue, and is the result of long and careful study, and for enriching and making blood will be found fully competent to do all for which it is represented. Weak and debilitate people who fear the approach of consumption from this cause, will find a friend in the Germ Syrup which will steer them clear of this dire complaint.

I do not mean to assert that it will cure consumption where the lungs are already attacked, established consumption cannot be cured, it may help them considerably by prolonging life, but it would not effect a cure. I am frequently asked by my correspondents how long the treatment should be continued. In reply I may say the time varies in accordance with the nature of the case. It should almost be regarded as a food-medicine. In ordinary cases eight weeks will produce remarkable results, and in numerous cases marked improvement follows the taking of the first bottle.

HERBAL PRESCRIPTIONS

The Germ Syrup is not unpleasant to the taste; it is a concentrated preparation, making the dose for an adult a teaspoonful in a half-wineglass full of cold water three times a day, either on the top of each meal or half an hour after each meal. Dose from 13 to 16 years of age, from half to three parts of a teaspoonful in a half-wineglass full of cold water three times a day; and reduced for youths accordingly.

I suggest that it be taken on the top of each meal, because it has to do its work along with the food, and in the next instance it would not be forgotten. The diet particulars as listed would greatly assist the Germ Syrup. It would be useless to give the prescription because it can only be made by a special process; were it only to mix or to boil I would willingly give it.

The Germ Syrup can always be taken with confidence, as nothing but good can attend its use. And if the patient be closely confined all day, and resides in the town, by all means try to get into the country a little in an evening, for to describe the value of pure air would fill a book. But I am not going to weary the patience of my reader with all its virtues; but if you want to weary the patience of the undertaker for an unlimited period the Germ Syrup and the country air should do it. Ask a friend to go with you for a ramble in the green fields. All this may seem a trouble at the beginning, but it will soon become a pleasure, and one you will look forward to. Don't, like the majority, be closely confined all day, then close yourself up in the house until bedtime, then close yourself up in a bedroom, breathing your own breath all night, which means looking for weakness and debility. The wise make an effort to keep health when in possession of it, rather than have to look for it when lost.

I suppose my reader will say, "How about the green fields in winter?" The fields in winter it may be necessary to abandon, but a sharp walk in a keen frosty air will be attended with similar beneficial results, and in many instances more so, because in most people it will create an appetite to be envied, and further, will in itself act as a tonic to the general system. Therefore everything is for good when rightly applied, and as I am strongly opposed to closed-up bedrooms, knowing too well the unthought-of mischief they create, I will now tell you how to ventilate a bedroom (in case you do not know) during the summer months, without fear of catching cold. Procure a piece of wood about two inches thick the exact width of the window frame, then lift up the bottom sash, fix in your piece of wood, and pull the sash down to it. Here you will find you have the window closed top and bottom, still the center is open two inches. This leaves nice play for fresh air, which directs itself up to the ceiling and distributes itself into the room, thus creating no draft whatever, but a gentle, continuous supply of fresh air. This may be resorted to in winter to the extent of about a half-inch, unless the weather is too severe; a little judgment is necessary.

I would suggest the bedroom door be left wide open also, in summer if not in winter, but not if there be a bed head in a direct line with the door and window. A bedroom fireplace should never be stopped up, it makes a good exit for foul air as the fresh air enters. And now if you will take a little notice of the rules I have laid down, and carry them out accordingly, the time is not far distant when good health will brighten the home of most of my readers. The Germ Syrup is 2 shillings per bottle, sent postage paid, and serves an adult 7 days; double quantity, 14 days' treatment, would be sent post paid for 3 shillings; an 8 weeks' course would be sent for 12 shillings, making a saving of 2 shillings for six days, besides saving stationery, time and postage. If for youths it serves double the time. The following is a list of constitutional ailments for which the Germ Syrup is adapted:

HERBAL PRESCRIPTIONS

Night Sweats,
Hysteria,
Extreme Weakness,
Constitutional Epilepsy,
Neurasthenia,
Asthmatic Bronchitis,
Hypochondria,
Asthma,
Nervous Debility (constitutional),
General Debility (constitutional),
Hoarseness and Wheezing,
Stomach Coughs,
Debility Coughs,
Coughs arising from the weakness of the bronchial tubes.

Progressive Consumption, where the lungs are not already diseased. Even then it should somewhat arrest decay, and accordingly prolong the life of the consumptive.

Capacity for study is developed, strength and energy take the place of weakness and depression.

GENERAL INFORMATION

Those who desire to have their prescription made up exactly as prescribed in this book should not take the book to the herbalist, take only a written copy of the prescription; by taking the book the herbalist sees the name of the ailment for which the prescription is intended, and in many instances, if short of one or two of the ingredients, or to save time and trouble is induced to use substitutes, regardless of the prescription submitted; of course this is all right if the same answers your purpose, but should the same fail, don't blame our prescription. Please note that we do not sell herbs, roots, or barks of any kind separately;

only combined in the form of a prescription. Neither do we sell herbs, roots, or barks to form prescriptions other than our own prescriptions. The three packets rate need not be confined to one kind, for family requirements three packets of any assorted kinds would be sent post-paid for 2 shillings.

Where pills are included in the prescription the pills are sent along with the herbs. I mention this because many people when ordering say, send on the herbs only, as I have some pills belonging to the last order; you cannot have too many of the herbal pills by you, no matter which kind, because they are always useful, even when not under the influence of the herbs, in fact many people (in mild cases) do not resort to the herbs, they take only the pills. We would send a shilling box of any of the pills named in this book (without the herbs), but we do not send the herbs without the pills, at least were we to do so the price would be the same. For convenience and quickness of dispatch the ingredients of each prescription (when ordered direct from us) are mixed one with the other, forming one complete packet, that is to say, the ingredients of one making are in one packet; of course if a person orders three lots he would receive three complete packets. The pills are in a pill box among the herbs for compactness. It is a wise proceeding for any person to occasionally assist nature with a harmless vegetable liver pill as described previously, or assist the stomach in performing its proper function by an occasional resort to digestives, or occasionally filter the kidneys with the pills named on prior, and in the spring and fall of the year purify the blood with a few packets of said prescription; by so doing you feel that life is worth living, because when the stomach, liver, kidneys, and the blood are in order the whole mechanism is in order at least constitutionally, and there is an old saying that "prevention is better than cure"; it is certainly less trouble. Many people are under the impression that anything in the form of a pill must necessarily be a purgative, this is not so, the only really aperient pill in this book is that on page 13. This pill is nice and mild in its action, and may be used in cases of Constipation in place of the Turkey Rhubarb referred to on page 30, and also for cleansing the kidneys. Price one shilling per box.

We cannot always dispatch goods on day of receipt of order; you may have to wait a day or two The same may be said of letters asking for advice. Always give your name and address in full and let it be plainly written.

Herbs do not taste so herby if instead of boiling you scald them in the same way as when you make tea, and those who prefer medicine sweet may with advantage add to each pint an ounce of licorice root, boil the licorice root in the water you are going to pour on the herbs. Roots and barks should always be boiled. It is not necessary to bottle the medicine, it may be kept in a jug if strained quite clear; it should be kept in a cold place or it is liable to ferment (turn sour) before it can be consumed. But with ordinary care and keeping to the doses it should keep. During the summer months the contents of the packet could be well mixed, then divided into two parts, and make only half quantity. If two or three persons are going to take it at the same time, you may safely venture to make the quart even in summer; this of course refers to where a quart is specified. Always scald out the vessel with boiling water before using it for a fresh supply. Inflammations, cramp, pleurisy, and fevers should have immediate attention, and be submitted to the care of a local doctor, in fact all acute or critical cases.

INDIGESTION

The following with many people is wonderful in counteracting acid and creating assimilation of the food, in numerous instances digesting food as if by magic; it is also possessed of great cleansing properties, is sweet, pleasant to the taste, and feeds the constitution; a wineglass full is more beneficial than the same quantity of port wine, and can be taken easily by people who do not like medicines of a bitter nature.

> Sassafras Bark ½ oz
> Guiacum Raspings ½ oz
> Mazereon root ½ oz
> Stillingia root ½ oz
> Arcticum Lappa ½ oz
> Sasparilla ½ oz
> Astralagus (root) 6 drachms

Boil slowly in a quart of water down to a pint, then strain, boil the same again in a pint of water 10 or 15 minutes, strain, and add to the other, when cold take a large wineglass full three times a day shortly after meals. This medicine must be kept in a cold place.

At meal times, eat slowly and do not overload your stomach. When taking this medicine for the purpose of cleansing the system double doses may be taken.

SMOKING AND DRINK HABIT

Although I am not of opinion that total abstinence from smoking is absolutely necessary to retain vitality, I have yet to learn how it can do any good, and to those who have not yet commenced the habit, my advice is do not begin; if you never begin you will never miss it.

To the confirmed smoker it would be difficult to describe what might be termed moderation, because one man may be able to smoke six pipes of tobacco daily with less effect than another man's three. But I say if you observe any unpleasant effect from smoking, the less you smoke the better; and if during the process of smoking you are continually spitting the less you smoke the better; but if a man spits little or none whilst smoking, and observes no unpleasant head sensations or depressing effect, I see no reason why he should not occasionally indulge the habit, the great principle being moderation.

The same rule applies to intoxicants. Excess can only terminate in emaciation and prostration of strength; see the confirmed drinker with his shaggy hair, his protruding eyes and his muddled brain; see the new beginner with his jaunty air, his rollicking gait, and his artificial hilarity, modesty has left him- vanity takes its place- hear him boasting how many drinks he can take; but see him the following morning before he's had the opportunity to revive the previous day's dissipation, then, reader, you may drop the curtain.

And yet intoxicants are good in many instances; a little whiskey with many people will assist digestion, and a half bottle of stout at bedtime to those not in the habit of drinking stout often (to the sleepless) induces sleep. But if your selection cannot be occasionally resorted to without danger of plunging into extremes, leave it alone entirely.

SUDDEN ILLNESS

When taken suddenly ill immediately send for a doctor, and in the meantime recline in a half erect position on the sofa or bed, and have a half-pint of equal parts milk and water boiled with as much powdered cayenne added as would cover a sixpence, drink this slowly with a teaspoon whilst hot; keep sipping it until the doctor arrives. If poisoning is suspected drink all the milk you can (without the water) until he comes. If your illness is attended with feverishness the following would be more suitable; a half-pint of boiling water poured on a pennyworth of saffron, make the same cool as quick as possible, and when about milk warm take a wineglass full, and every ten minutes afterwards a tablespoonful until the doctor comes.

TONIC

A simple but valuable tonic when not particularly ailing, but feeling somewhat played out, is made as follows

Tincture of Gentian 2 drachms
Tincture of Chinchona 2 drachms
Tinctiu^e of Cayenne 20 drops

Water to 8 oz. and take a tablespoonful three times a day. Obtainable at any herbalists, or we will send it post paid (water to add when you receive it), for 12 penny stamps, double quantity is 2 shillings.

BABIES, CHILDREN, AND SPECTACLES

Any person who remembers candle-light days will also remember that they seldom saw either a child or youth wearing spectacles. The impaired vision of children of the present day is caused principally through thoughtlessness of mothers and nurses; the mother dills baby in her lap and allows it to gaze to its heart's content at the gas light crooning to it "does e ickle babsy wabsy like e bo bell." The mother who can afford a bassinet takes particular care to line the interior of the bassinet and the interior of the hood with pure white, little babsy whichever way it looks has its eyes fixed on about the last thing capable of resting its sight; and there is also that little white cot, when you have that little white cot fixed up with white hood and white curtains, be kind enough, for baby's sake, to fix the cot with the gas light behind it. And allow me to inform you that the two best shades for the lining of the cot and bassinet are black or dark green, and if you do not want to see your baby sooner or later wearing spectacles you will do well to remember this.

And let your final instructions to nurse be that when she reaches the form in the park, with that nice novelette, to take particular care to keep the child's back to the sun, babies are attracted by the sun or gas light, and either can pave the way for irreparable mischief to the sight.

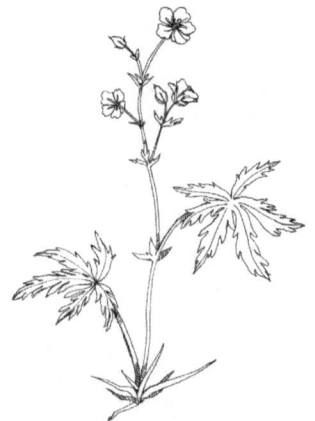

Cranesbill

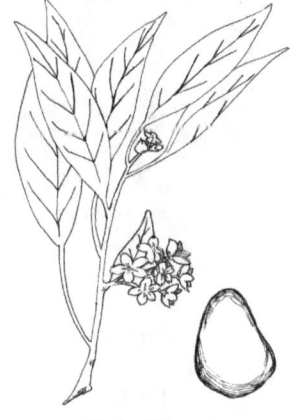

Cola Plant

HERBAL PRESCRIPTIONS

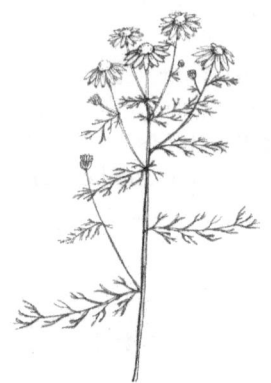

Chamomile

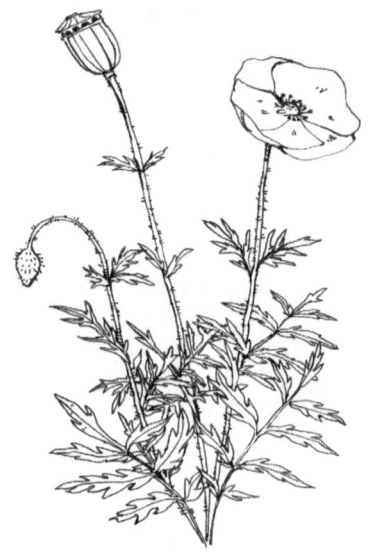

Poppy

END